Youth Diet's Impact on Body Fat

Abella k

Author: Abella k

Title: Youth Diet's Impact on Body Fat

This book is a product of [Publisher's Abella k

ISBN:

Relationship Between Youth Diet and Body

FatAim: The purpose of this book was to look at the differences in fat-related diet habits of college students of varying BMI statuses and sex at a large mid-western public University.

Sample: It was a quantitative study with cross-sectional design. Convenient sampling was used.

Materials: An online survey was conducted via filling out a fat-related diet habits questionnaire.

Statistical analysis: Demographic data was summarized and presented in table of distribution frequencies, mean and standard deviations. To test the hypotheses, multifactorial two-way ANOVA was used for the main part of the questionnaire. Any p-value ≤ 0.05 was considered significant.

Outcomes: The p-values of the summary scores for sex, and different BMI categories was 0.48 and 0.31 respectively. The scores fell between "often" and "sometimes". Similar patterns were observed between males and females and varying BMI categories. There were no significant differences found in the fat-related diet habits between sex and varying BMI statuses.

Conclusion: This study demonstrated that no differences were observed between fat-related diet habits of college students between males and females, and between varying BMI statuses. However, it also provides evidence of improvement in the nutritional status and dietary habits, especially fat consumption of young adults.

TABLE OF CONTENTS

Page

CHAPTER I

INTRODUCTION

Over the decades, obesity continues to be a major public health concern around the globe and specifically in the U.S. Obesity is a preventable condition, however, there is a pre-dominant obesogenic environment characterized by an unlimited supply of energy-dense, highly palatable convenient foods at a low price (Freedman & Brochado, 2010). According to a report from 1998-2008, more than 68% of the U.S. adults were overweight, and 35% were obese (Flegal, Caroll, Ogden, & Curtin, 2010). This poses severe health risks and a huge economic burden on society because overweight and obesity lead to chronic diseases such as hypertension, type 2 diabetes, cardiovascular diseases, cancer and premature death (Report of a joint WHO/FAO expert consultation, 2003).

Monitoring the fat intake during the transition from adolescence to young adulthood is crucial because it is found to be challenging period, there are many lifestyle and dietary changes involved (Lassi, Moin, & Bhutta, 2017). There is often increased consumption of fast-foods and processed foods and decreased consumption of fruits and vegetables because they start making independent food choices (Neumark-Sztainer et al., 2011). There are nationally recognized guidelines given by The Academy of Nutrition and Dietetics for grains, protein, fruits, vegetables, dairy, fats/oils, added sugars, and physical activity, despite the available guidelines, nutritional problems continue to be prevalent in college students (U.S Department of Health and Human Services, Centers for Disease Control and Prevention, 2019).

The recommendations for oils in a 2000Kcal healthy diet is 27g, about 5 teaspoons. Around 20%-35% of the total calories should come from fats is the recommendation. The average intake of oils in the US by young adults is 35-40g per day (U.S. Department of Health and Human Services, Centers for Disease Control and Prevention, 2019). Saturated fats (SF) should account for no more than 10% of the total calories. Some common sources of SF in the American diet are burgers, sandwiches, pizza, taco, rice, pasta, meat, poultry, seafood dishes (U.S. Department of Health and Human Services, Centers for Disease Control and Prevention, 2019). It is very important to monitor the fat intake because as per the latest dietary guidelines and current pattern in the U.S., college students consume more than the recommended intake for saturated fats (U.S. Department of Health and Human Services, Centers for Disease Control and Prevention, 2019).

Their food choices are influenced by a number of factors including taste, cost, nutritive value, convenience, palatability and weight issues (Glanz, Basil, Maibach, Goldberg, & Snyder, 1998), stress (Zellnar, Saito, & Gonzalez, 2007), living condition (Freedman, 2010), lack of access to the food preparation facilities (LaCaille, Dauner, Krambeer, & Pederson, 2011), poor nutrition education (Vidgen & Gallegos, 2014), campus food outlets (Niemeier, Raynor, Lloyd-Richardson, Rogers, & Wing, 2006), peer influence (Munt, Patridge, & Allman-Farinelli, 2017), and social media (Freeland-Graves & Nitzke, 2013). Portion sizes have also shown to affect weight because restaurants serve large portion sizes for fatty foods (Diliberti, Bordi, Conklin, Roe, & Rolls, 2004). Physical activity is another important factor influencing obesity. More than 60% of college students do not engage in moderate or vigorous exercise (National College Health Assessment 2: Reference Group Executive Summary 2011).

There have also been differences observed in the dietary habits between male and female university students. Male students were found to have less-healthful eating habits as compared to females. They consumed fast foods frequently (Huang, Song, Schemmel, & Hoerr, 1994), were less likely to read the nutrition labels (Oakes & Slotterback, 2000), have breakfast, and prepare their own food (Musingo & Wang, 2009). A survey-based study reported that male students consumed more fat than female students while female's diet consisted less of fibers, fruits and vegetables. Also, female students were found to engage more in healthful eating practices (Li et al., 2012).

Various interventions have been conducted in the past in the effort to improve the nutrition knowledge and behavior of college students some of which include in-person interaction, online or through Point-Of-Purchase (POP) messages. Nutrition course (Ha & Caine-Bish, 2011), cooking demonstrations (Levy & Auld, 2004), and use of traffic light labels (Thorndike, Sonnenberg, Riis, Barraclough, & Levy, 2012) were some of the interventions found effective in improving their nutrition knowledge as well as food choices. BMI (Body Mass Index) is a useful tool to measure overweight and obesity. It is an estimate of the fat mass in the body. The higher the BMI, the higher is the risk of chronic diseases. There have been constant increases in weight and BMI during college life and hence, it is very important to monitor the BMI during young adulthood coupled with the fat intake (Gropper, Simmons, Connell, & Ulrich, 2012).

Statement of the Problem

Over the years, there has been an increase in obesity rates in the U.S. In 2015-2016 data reports, about 39.6% of the American adults over the age of 20 years were obese. Also, obesity in young adults was found to be 18.5%. Boys were more likely to be obese than girls (Hales, Caroll, Fryar, & Ogden, 2017). There is a significant change in the dietary habits reported in the first year of college and these habits are likely to continue throughout their life (Neumark-Sztainer et al., 2011). High saturated fat intake and low intake of fruits and vegetables is observed among college students. Regular consumption of high-fat foods poses them a risk of developing obesity, diabetes, hypertension, cardiovascular diseases and even cancer in the later years of life. However, college students do not find the need to modify their eating behaviors and they continue to consume foods high in fat and sugar (Neumark-Sztainer et al., 2011).

Consumption of fat and BMI status are co-related to each other, there is continuous increase in BMI status and weight throughout the four years of college coupled with high intake of fatty foods (Gropper et al., 2012). Higher consumption of fat has been noted in the individuals with higher BMI statuses. Fat consumption also varies with sex among college students (Li et al., 2012). However, not enough studies have been done to observe the dietary patterns of college students, especially including the differences in sex as well as the four BMI categories. This study examines their fat-related dietary habits with respect to sex and varying BMI statuses. This will give the researchers an idea about the current fat-related eating habits of college students and it will help the researchers to develop strategies to monitor their BMI, educate them and will contribute to the existing pool of research.

Purpose Statement

The objective of this study was to examine the differences in fat-related diet habits in college students of varying BMI statuses and sex at a large mid-western public university.

Hypotheses

1. There were differences in fat-related diet habits in college students of varying BMI statuses at a large mid-western public university.
2. There were differences in fat-related diet habits in college students of different sex at a large mid-western public university.

Operational Definitions

- College student: someone who is between 18-25 years in age and enrolled at Kent State University Main Campus
- BMI classification/statuses (kg/m^2): It is calculated as: (weight in kg/(height in meter)^2) and is classified as: Underweight (<18.5), normal (18.5 - <25), overweight (25 - <30), obese (≥30)

- Fat-related diet habits: The frequency of consumption of foods that have relatively high fat content. This includes full-fat products, visible fat, fried foods, fat-rich desserts and sweets, etc.

CHAPTER II

LITERATURE REVIEW

Fats and Oils

Fat or lipid is one of the three important macronutrients found in both plants and animals in varying amounts. The primary source of energy is carbohydrates. However, in its deficit, fat provides the required energy to the body. It also has other essential functions in the body such as insulation, lubricants, storage and is involved highly in metabolism. Acylglycerols are the major lipids in the body. Around 85% of the energy is stored in the form of Triacylglycerols (TAG) and is involved in metabolism as a primary source of energy (Stipanuk, 2006).

Fatty acids (FA) are the building blocks of fat and there are different types of fat made up by a combination of fatty acids, Poly-unsaturated (PUFA), mono-unsaturated (MUFA), saturated fats (SF) and trans fats (TF) in different amounts. For example, oil is composed mostly of unsaturated fatty acids and a little of the saturated fatty acid while butter contains more saturated fat and lesser amounts of PUFA and MUFA (U.S. department of Health and Human Services, Centers for Disease Control and Prevention, 2019).

- PUFA: They are mostly liquid at room temperature. Good sources of omega-6 FA include walnut, pecans, sunflower, cottonseed, corn and soybean oils. An important type of PUFA- omega-3 FA is found in soybean, flaxseeds, and fish such as Tuna, Mackerel, Herring, Salmon, Trout (Stipanuk, 2006).

- MUFA: They are mostly liquid at room temperature. They are found most abundantly in olive, canola and peanut oils. Other sources in which they are less abundant are peanuts, avocado, and other nuts. It is also a part of animal foods such as chicken, pork, lamb, beef (U.S. department of Health and Human Services, Centers for Disease Control and Prevention, 2019).
- SF: They are mostly solid at room temperature. They are found in large amounts in coconut oil, beef fat, butter, cheese, palm kernel oil, pork, and chicken fats. It is also found in plant sources like nuts (U.S. department of Health and Human Services, Centers for Disease Control and Prevention, 2019).
- TF: They are mostly solid at room temperature. They are unsaturated FA differing in structure and health effects from other unsaturated FA. Trans fats are usually produced in partially hydrogenated vegetable oils and ruminant fats (U.S. department of Health and Human Services, Centers for Disease Control and Prevention, 2019). Trans fats are known to be atherogenic by stimulating a rise in cholesterol levels (Stipanuk, 2006).

Types and Effects of Fatty Acids in the Body

Fatty acids are of two types, essential and non-essential fatty acids. Non-essential fatty acids can be produced in the body while essential fatty acids are those that are not produced in the body and should be included in the diet to fulfill the requirement. Some of the MUFA and PUFA have shown a positive effect on reducing the risk of chronic diseases. Olive oil is rich in MUFA and is shown to reduce chronic disease risk such as cardiovascular diseases. Alpha-linolenic acid, which is an omega-3 fatty acid, is also included in good fats and is present in plant-based foods like canola oil, olive oil, flaxseed and nuts as well as animal fats. Consumption of fish and fish products rich in omega-3 FA has been shown to have a protective effect against CVD (cardiovascular diseases), depression, cataract, immune function diseases and cancer (Stipanuk, 2006).

Metabolism of Lipid

The breakdown of lipid results into its basic form, free fatty acids (FFA). FFAs are rapidly mobilized. In starvation state, they are used up by the cells, while in fed state, they are stored as triacylglycerols (TAG). TAG is further transported from the intestine in chylomicrons and from the liver in VLDL to the extrahepatic tissues. The liver plays an essential role in the metabolism of lipid as it facilitates the digestion and absorption of the lipid by the production of bile, it is involved in lipid synthesis as well as oxidation, and it also plays an integral part in the synthesis and metabolism of lipoproteins (Rodwell, Bender, Kennely, Botham, & Weil, 2015). Fat absorbed from the diet and lipid synthesized by the liver and adipose tissue is transported to different tissues and organs for utilization and storage. Since lipids are insoluble in water, they are transported packed in lipoproteins. There are four major lipoproteins involved in the transport of lipid: low-density lipoprotein (LDL), high-density lipoprotein (HDL), chylomicrons and very low-density lipoprotein (VLDL). They are inter-converted as per the needs and state of the body (fed state and fasting state) and are tightly controlled.

If there is an accumulation of LDL, VLDL and/or cholesteryl esters in the arteries, it could result into fatty plaques blocking the vessels. Common food sources of cholesterol include meat, poultry, and fish fats, eggs, dairy fats (Stipanuk, 2006). Synthesis and disposal of cholesterol must be tightly regulated to meet the required amount by the body and preventing its accumulation at the same time. The accumulation of cholesterol into coronary arteries eventually leads to atherosclerosis and CVDs (Stipanuk, 2006).

Fat Consumption and Risk for Chronic Diseases

Excess visceral fat is known to be the major factor for causing all the disorders related to metabolism, including Chronic Kidney Disease (CKD) (Tchernof & Després, 2013). According to the past research, there is a clear association found between BMI and visceral obesity which in turn is a risk factor of other diseases (Hsu, McCulloch, Iribarren, Darbinian, & Go, 2006). According to the CDC (Centers for Disease Control and prevention) report, about 15% of the U.S. adults are estimated to have CKD. It is found to be more common in women as compared to men (U.S. Department of Health and Human Services, Centers for Disease Control and Prevention, 2019). Data from the Framingham Heart Study Offspring Cohort showed a 68% relative increase in the odds of developing CKD in individuals with BMI over 30 compared to those with normal weight. However, after adjusting for variables, the relationship was no longer significant (Foster et al., 2008). Another study involving 11,000 healthy men followed for 14 years, higher BMI was associated with an increased risk of CKD (Gelber et al., 2005).

Hypertension is another concern for the population at risk or already having high consumption of fat. Studies have shown that weight gain raises blood pressure (Hall, Crook, Jones, Wofford, & Dubbert, 2002), weight loss lowers blood pressure (Jones et al., 2012) and excess weight gain is a good indicator of hypertension (Hall et al., 2010). Previous research on animals demonstrated that there was a consistent rise in blood pressure with excess weight gain induced by a prolonged high-fat diet (Dobrian, Davies, Prewitt, & Lauterio, 2000). Clinical studies also suggest that uncontrolled weight gain is a crucial contributor to elevated blood pressure in patients with primary hypertension. Further, weight loss of only 5%-10% lowered blood pressure in subjects with normal as well as those with hypertension (Jones, 1999). Research conducted on populations from around the world showed a strong association between weight gain and hypertension (Cooper, rotimi, & ward, 1999).

Western diet, which is the typical diet common in Northern Europe and the U.S. has been reported as a risk factor for depression. it also included the replacement of PUFA and MUFA with SF (Jacka et al., 2010). On the contrary, a higher adherence to the Mediterranean diet rich in legumes, fruits, vegetables, fish, and cereals but low in meat and dairy products was inversely associated with the risk of depression (Sánchez-Villegas et al., 2009). According to the result of a prospective cohort study, an inverse association between olive oil consumption and depression was found, however, after the adjustments for the variables, the relationship was attenuated (Sánchez-Villegas et al., 2011).

Studies have also shown the association of a high-fat diet with an increased risk for autoimmune diseases (Manzel et al., 2014). Multiple Sclerosis (MS) incidence may be positively associated with the consumption of animal fat (Esparza, Sasaki, & Kesteloot, 1995) and meat (Lauer, 1994) and also obesity while diets high in PUFA and plant fiber may decrease MS risk (Agranoff, Bernard, & Goldberg, 1974). Further, a retrospective study suggested that high BMI and obesity before adulthood were linked to a higher risk of developing MS (Munger, Chitnis, & Ascherio, 2009). Several case-controlled studies strongly linked obesity and metabolic syndrome to Psoriasis (Sterry, Stober, & Menter, 2007) and Rheumatoid Arthritis (Ferraz-Amaro, González-Juanatey, López-Mejias, Riancho-Zarrabeitia, & González-Gay, 2013). In general, obesity and metabolic syndrome predispose individuals to a plethora of diseases including autoimmune diseases (Manzel et al., 2014).

Cardiovascular Diseases

CVD is widely recognized as the leading cause of premature death in both, developed and developing countries (Xu et al., 2012). Low diet quality and less physical activity increase their risk of chronic diseases according to the research in the previous years (Forshee et al., 2006). More than 60% of college students do not engage in moderate or vigorous exercise according to a report issued by the American College Health Association in 2011 (National College Health Assessment, 2011). Research involving adolescents and young adults demonstrated that body composition factors like waist-hip ratio, body fatness and dietary factors such as sugar-sweetened beverages, saturated fat, MUFA, alcohol intake were significant indicators of coronary heart disease (CHD) risk (Mansfield, McPherson, & Koski, 1999).

A study performed at Rhode Island University on first-year college students revealed that healthy dietary trends were significantly associated with lower TAG, glucose, weight circumference and higher level of HDL (High-Density Lipoprotein). Also, higher consumption of fiber, lower consumption of sugar, saccharine and alcohol was associated with decreased risk of CHD. Lastly, BMI was more strongly related to CHD risk factors (Fernandes, Arts, Dimond, Hirshberg, & Lofgren, 2013). Although college students indicated that they were aware of the risk factors, their behaviors did not reflect their nutrition knowledge (Fernandes et al., 2013).

The type of fat has been considered more important than the amount of the fat for the reduction of CVD and death (Elosua, Marrugat, Molina, Pons, & Pujol, 1994). CVD risk can be reduced by decreasing the amount of SFA and replacing it with PUFA and MUFA in the diet (Hu et al., 2001). In a study conducted on the population at risk for CVD, it was found that the subjects with a high intake of total fat, SFA and trans-fat were less physically active and had a higher incidence of Diabetes. They also consumed less fiber and carbohydrates, and more cholesterol. PUFAs and MUFAs were inversely related to the risk of CVD while SFAs were associated with increased risk (PREDIMED Study Investigators, 2015).

High-fat and low-carbohydrates diet may cause nutritional deficiencies because of long-term changes in the plasma substrates (Marshall, Bessessen, & Hamman, 1997). It causes alterations in carbohydrate and fat metabolism, increasing circulating glucose, Free Fatty Acids (FFA) and causing insulin resistance (Bisschop et al., 2001).

Epidemiological studies have shown cognitive deficits after chronic ingestion of high-fat diets (Zhang, Mckeown, Muldoon, & Tang, 2006).

High fat intake has been associated with a greater risk of developing Alzheimer's disease (Ortega et al., 1997). A study conducted with a short-term high-fat, low-carbohydrate diet, led to increasing the circulating FFA concentrations and decreased cognition in healthy subjects. It showed that such diets could be detrimental to the heart and brain (Holloway et al., 2011). Besides, a high total cholesterol level is strongly associated with Coronary Artery Disease (CAD). Its accumulation coupled with high plasma levels of LDL has found to be a significant risk factor for atherosclerosis whereas adequate levels of HDL has been linked to reduced risk of atherosclerosis (Stipanuk, 2006).

Previous research shows that three factors are playing important roles in the etiology of atherosclerosis and CVD: oxidative stress (Yokoyama, 2004), lipid abnormalities (Castelli, 1986) and chronic inflammation (Hansson, 2005). The result of the study conducted on rodents demonstrated that the supplementation of flaxseed oil and alpha-Lipoic acid might contribute to prevent atherogenesis and then decrease the incidence of CVD (Xu et al., 2012). Research shows that replacing SF with unsaturated fats significantly reduced the risk of cardiovascular diseases (CVD), reduce blood levels of triglycerides (TG) and low-density lipoprotein (LDL). Trans fats are also to be consumed in very limited amounts because they have been shown to increase the risk of CVD and partly LDL (Stipanuk, 2006).

Diabetes

Food and beverages rich in energy, fat, and sugar are recognized as the major factors for obesogenic environments in humans (Nolan, Damm, & Prentki, 2011). Because fat is energy-dense, fat intake may play an important role in the development of type 2 diabetes (T2D) (Lottenberg, Afonso, Lavrador, Machado, & Nakandakare, 2012). Prolonged consumption of a western diet rich in sugar and saturated fat has been thought to play an important role in the development of type 2 diabetes (van Dam, Willett, Rimm, Stampfer, & Hu, 2002). The administration of a high-fat diet (HFD) for two months to rats was found a fast and easy way to induce metabolic syndrome and oxidative disorders without modulation of glycemia (Auberval et al., 2014). Epidemiological studies also showed that a diet rich in fat and sugar was a greater risk factor than either of them (Basu, Yoffe, Hills, Lustig, & Wagner, 2013). The combination of high fat and fructose in the diet of rats allowed the development of diabetes, insulin resistance and dyslipidemia (Lozano et al., 2016).

Chronic insulin resistance comprises not only impaired muscle insulin action but also increased rates of gluconeogenesis in obese and diabetic patients (Gastaldelli et al., 2000). Moreover, this type of diet was also found to be associated with diabetes-related complications such as hepatic steatosis (Lozano et al., 2016). In a study including both humans and mice, a single oral dose of saturated fat was found enough to increase hepatic triglyceride (TG) accumulations, insulin resistance, gluconeogenesis and ATP (Adenosine Triphosphate) concentrations in the human liver and similar results were observed in mice (Hernández et al., 2017).

Evidence from lifestyle interventions indicated that reduced consumption of total and saturated fat in combination with high fiber intake and physical activity prevent the risk of developing T2D in individuals with impaired glucose metabolism (Penn et al., 2013). Plant sources of fat were found to be a better choice as compared to animal fats (Parillo & Riccardi, 2004) and high meat/meat products consumptions showed a positive association with the risk of T2D (Micha, Wallace, & Mozaffarian, 2010). Also, fatty fish ("For the InterAct Consortium, The Prospective Association between Total and Type of Fish Intake and Type 2 Diabetes in 8 European Countries: EPIC-InterAct Study.", 2012), intakes and blood concentrations of PUFAs (Alhazmi, Stojanovski, McEvoy, & Garg, 2014), alpha-linolenic acid (Wu et al., 2012), long-chain fish n-3 PUFA from foods (Villegas et al., 2011) were inversely associated with T2D risk. On the contrary, other studies showed no indication of the inverse relationship (Djoussé, Gaziano, Buring, & Lee, 2011).

Cancer

Consumption of dietary fat has been linked to gastric cancer risk. Gastric cancer is one of the most common malignant tumors worldwide, especially in developing countries (Jemal et al., 2011). Previous research has shown that dietary factors play an important role in the etiology of gastric cancer (Parkin, 2006). Consumption of salty foods (Ge et al., 2012), red and processed meat(Zhu et al., 2013), preserved food is thought to increase gastric cancer risk while intake of fruits, vegetables (Freedman et al., 2008), and antioxidant vitamins (Zhou, Wang, Meng, & Zhai, 2016) have been shown to reduce the risk. Dietary fat has been reported to be related to various malignant tumors such as breast (Thiebaut et al., 2007), colorectal (Butler et al., 2009), pancreatic, and prostate cancers (Arem et al., 2013).

A meta-analysis done on observational studies demonstrated a positive association between the intake of saturated fats and gastric cancer risk, and an inverse relation between the intake of PUFAs, vegetable consumption to gastric cancer risk (Han et al., 2015). Many experimental studies have also shown that a high intake of saturated fat could increase the risk of breast and colorectal cancers (Escrich, Moral, Grau, Costa, & Solanas, 2007).

Mediterranean diet rich in olive oil has been linked to having a protective effect against cancer (Trichopoulou, Lagiou, Kuper, & Trichopoulos, 2000) A cohort study also found that adherence to the Mediterranean diet reduced the risk of gastric cancer significantly (Buckland et al., 2010). However, some case-control studies also showed null and even inverse relation between dietary fat and gastric cancer risk, hence, more research is needed to understand the relation, if any (Arem et al., 2013).

Cholesterol has been linked to increased risk of many diseases because its accumulation in the bloodstream can cause atherosclerotic plaques which can cause coronary artery disease (Satoh et al., 2010). A cancer prevention cohort study showed that higher concentrations of HDL were associated with decreased risk of lung cancer, and liver cancer (Ahn et al., 2009). In relation to dietary cholesterol and cancer risk, there have been studies showing elevated risk of colorectal, pancreas, and kidney cancers, while other studies showed no association with cancers of stomach (Lucenteforte et al.,

2009), pancreas (Lucenteforte et al., 2009), ovary (Bidoli et al., 2002), prostate (Bidoli et al., 2002), and kidney (Allen et al., 2009).

In a large study conducted in Canada, it was found that the total cholesterol intake was associated with increased risk of cancers of stomach, colon, rectum, pancreas, lung, breast, kidney, bladder. A negative correlation was observed with prostate cancer and no association was found for testis, ovary, and brain (Hu et al., 2012). Interestingly, one of the cohort studies also found that a combination of iron and cholesterol in the blood above 75th percentile significantly increased risk of all cancers supporting the theory that iron-induced oxidation of serum lipids play a crucial role in the etiology of cancer (Wells, Mainous, Everett, & Gill, 2005).

Obesity

Over the decades, obesity continues to be a major public health concern around the globe and specifically in the U.S. Obesity is a preventable condition, however, there is a pre-dominant obesogenic environment characterized by an unlimited supply of energy-dense, highly palatable convenient foods at a low price (Freedman & Brochado, 2010). This is coupled with an incline in the sedentary lifestyle of the population which further increases the incidence and prevalence of obesity (Freedman & Brochado, 2010). According to a report from 1998-2008, more than 68% of the U.S. adults were overweight, and 35% were obese (Flegal et al., 2010).

Incidence and Energy Balance

According to the NCHS data 2015-2016 for obesity, pre-school aged children had more prevalence of obesity than adolescents (12-19 years). From 1999-2000 through 2015-2016, a significant increase in the prevalence of obesity was observed in both youth and adults (Hales et al., 2017). This poses severe health risks and a huge economic burden on society because overweight and obesity lead to chronic diseases such as hypertension, type 2 diabetes, cardiovascular diseases, cancer and premature death (Report of joint WHO/FAO expert consultation, 2003). The etiology of obesity is highly complex and involves genetic, psychological, environmental, physiological, social, economic, and political factors that interact in varying degrees to contribute to the risk of developing obesity (Aronne et al., 2009). Young adults in Western countries are gaining weight faster than their parents and are more likely to gain weight than any other age (Allman-Farinelli, Chey, Bauman, Gill, & James, 2007).

Energy balance is defined as a condition in which energy intake is equivalent to the energy expenditure over the time period of observation. When energy intake exceeds the energy expenditure, the balance is positive and net body energy gain occurs which usually 60%-80% body fat (Hill & Commeford, 1996). Conversely, when energy expenditure exceeds the intake, there is negative energy balance and energy deficit occurs. A sedentary lifestyle and excess intake of calories contribute to overweight and obesity. Also, a continuous decline in physical activity has been observed between ages 18-29 years (Casperson, Pereira, & Curran, 2000).

Body Mass Index (BMI) and Weight

BMI is a useful measure of overweight and obesity. It is an estimate of your body fat and a good tool to estimate the risk of diseases that can occur with more body fat. BMI can be a useful tool to classify individuals as underweight, normal, overweight or obese. The higher your BMI, the more risk one has of diseases like heart diseases, high blood pressure, type 2 diabetes, breathing problems, and certain cancers. However, by itself, it is not indicative of overweight or obesity, a person could be overweight without having excess fat if the extra weight comes from the muscles, bones or body water. In contrast, the elderly population could fall into the normal BMI category with significant losses in body mass and reduced nutritional reserves. Moreover, genetic factors could be one of the causes for obesity risk. Studies on identical twins raised in different environments showed similar changes in body composition. Mutations in genes have been associated with early-onset and severe obesity in humans (Stipanuk, 2006).

In a study examining 131 students' weight over four years of college, they found that there were significant gains in weight, percent body fat and BMI (Gropper et al., 2012). Another study monitored the students' changes in weight, BMI, exercise frequency, and dietary patterns and it was found that they gained an average of 2.5kg in four years and met neither dietary guidelines nor physical activity recommendations (Racette, Deusinger, Strube, Highstein, & Deusinger, 2005). Research conducted in 2012 used anthropometric assessments and questionnaires to examine the weight trajectory of the students over the four years. There was a significant increase in weight and BMI over the four years and FFQ (Food Frequency Questionnaire) data showed that mean fruit and vegetable consumption was below the recommended intake for young adults. Also, the prevalence of overweight and obesity increased significantly from the beginning of freshman year to the end of senior year (Pope, Hansen, & Harvey, 2016).

The energy density of the foods is one of the determinants affecting the BMI of an individual. Energy-dense foods cause passive over-eating in terms of energy. They are usually high in fat and sugar but low in fiber and water (Rolls, 2009). Research showed that there was weight reduction with low energy-dense foods consumption (Ello-Martin, Roe, Ledikwe, Beach, & Rolls, 2007) while long-term studies showed a positive association of high energy-dense foods with weight gain (Savage, Marini, & Birch, 2008). Fruits and vegetables are rich in fiber, and antioxidants, therefore, are associated with weight control. According to a study, a diet rich in fruits and vegetables was generally found to be effective in preventing weight gain (He et al., 2004). Portion sizes have shown to affect weight because restaurants serve large portion sizes for fatty foods (Diliberti et al., 2004). In this environment, unlimited access to all-you-can-eat buffets and large portion sizes have been linked to weight gain (Levitsky, Halbmaier, & Mrdjenovic, 2004). One study conducted in a laboratory setting reported that reducing portion sizes affected the subjects' energy intake (Rolls, 2003). Another study conducted at San Jose University showed that portion sizes could be reduced resulting in equivalent reduction in the energy intake (Freedman & Brochado, 2010). Large portion sizes could also be replaced for low nutrient-dense foods like fruits and vegetables which can be protective against weight gain (Rolls, 2003).

Dietary Patterns of College Students

A study performed at Washington University showed that about 70% of the students observed weight gain in the first two years of their college. It also showed that many students did not consume enough fruits and vegetables and consumed fried and fast foods without any limitation (Racette et al., 2005). Young adults have shown to have the highest consumption of sugar-sweetened beverages (Kit, Fakhouri, Park, Nielsen, & Ogden, 2013), and poorest consumption of vegetables (Australian Health Survey: First Results, 2014–15, 2012). They also have the highest range of binge drinking, and these calories when not compensated, leads to weight gain (Nanney et al., 2015).

Increased consumption of ultra-processed foods and beverages such as soda, carbonated, and sugar-sweetened beverages have been considered as one of the contributors to obesity (Report of joint World Health Organization/Food and Agriculture Organization expert consultation, 2003). A cohort study showed that about 50% of the daily caloric intake of the participants at 23 years of age included ultra-processed foods (Bielemann, Motta, Minten, Horta, & Gingante, 2015). Studies specific to college students showed that most of them consumed at least one fast-food meal a week (Gerend, 2009), and some consumed as many as 6-8 meals (Driskell et al., 2005). Besides, college students consumed fast-food 70% more often as compared to non-college going students (Krukowski, Harvey-Berino, Kolodinsky, Narsana, & DeSisto, 2006). A typical fast-food meal contains more than 800 calories (Block et al., 2013), which for most adults, exceeds 30% of their daily calorie requirements (Urban et al., 2013). It was also found that the number of fast-food restaurants within a 0.5-mile radius of a person's home was positively correlated with the number of meals the person consumed there (Boone-Heinonen, 2011).

Besides, eating outside the home may be a determinant of obesity because foods served at restaurants are often high in fat and energy contents as compared to food prepared at home (Zoumas-Morse, Rock, Sobo, & Neuhouser, 2001). Number of processed food items typically high in sugar, fat, and sodium are available in grocery stores, mini-marts, and convenience stores. These products are heavily marketed not only to adults, but also children (Rolls, 2003). Not all fats are alike, hence the type of fat consumed should be considered. Previous research has established the useful effects of polyunsaturated fatty acids, mono-unsaturated fatty acids and harmful effects of consuming trans fats and saturated fatty acids (Hu, Manson, & Willett, 2001).

Physical activity

The most dramatic declines in physical activity has been observed during the transition from late adolescence to early adulthood (Gordon-Larsen, Nelson, & Popkin, 2004). A public weight gain prevention program needs only small changes in energy intake and physical activity. One program based on the concept of eating 100 kcal less per day and walking 2000 steps each day was found effective in increasing physical activity, reducing energy intake and reducing energy density (Stroebele et al., 2009) Food restriction is the most common strategy for treating obesity followed by the population (Wadden, 1993). However, individuals who were successful in achieving long-term weight loss maintenance were found to engage in high amounts of physical activity and not just calorie restriction (Wing & Hill, 2001). Most people consume high amounts of energy and very low energy expenditure. An increase in physical activity has been linked to restore and maintain the energy balance (Hill, Wyatt, & Peters, 2012).

Physical activity is an important determinant for developing an increased risk for obesity. The results from a Canadian representative sample data showed that 85% of the adults did not meet the minimum requirement of 150 minutes of moderate to vigorous physical activity every week (Colley et al., 2011). A more recent study also supported the declines in physical activity during this period (Kwan, Cairney, Faulkner, & Pullenayegum, 2012). Involvement in large amount of sedentary behaviors or sitting has been associated with multiple health problems like impaired lipid profile, greater energy intake, increased waist circumferences, and greater mortality risk (Colley et al., 2011).

Nutrition During Early Adulthood

The transition from adolescence to young adulthood could be challenging period because there are many lifestyle and dietary changes involved. Research showed that college students became more independent in making food choices and were likely to be affected by their peers which in turn led to unhealthy choices of foods (Lassi et al., 2017). There is often increased consumption of fast-foods and processed foods and decreased consumption of fruits and vegetables because they start making independent food choices (Neumark-Sztainer et al., 2011). These fast-foods are energy-dense, high in sugar and fat which could pose the risk of various diseases and conditions (Neumark-Sztainer et al., 2011). Their choices were also influenced by environmental factors like living condition, parental diet, nutrition education, and knowledge of the mother (Moreno et al., 2008). Other factors affecting their dietary choices were portion sizes, frequency of family dinners, and meal skipping (Moreno-Gómez et al., 2012).

There are nationally recognized guidelines given by The Academy of Nutrition and Dietetics for grains (6 ounce equivalents/day), dairy (3 cup equivalents/day), protein (5.5 ounce equivalents/day), fats/oils (five teaspoons/day), fruits (2 cup equivalents/day) and vegetables (2.5 cup equivalents/day), added sugars (limit to less than 10% of the total calories per day) to be consumed, and the amount of physical activity required (at least150 minutes of exercise each week (U.S. Department of Health and Human Services, Centers for Disease Control and Prevention, 2019). Despite the available guidelines, nutritional problems continue to be prevalent in college students. Adolescents described healthy foods as "natural stuff" or "home-grown vegetables". Almost no one mentioned about dairy in their opinions in one of the studies (Croll, Neumark-Sztainer, & Story, 2011). Many mentioned chips, cold-drinks, cola, candy, pizza, pies, cookies, peanut butter as unhealthy foods. However, they pointed out that unhealthy foods were conveniently available and more appealing. Interestingly, many students linked healthy foods to family dinners and relatives and less with friends and their peers. They realized that they consumed unhealthy foods, but they did it anyway. Another highlighting factor was that rarely did anyone mention about the food guide. Further, only a few were able to recognize the long-term benefits of following a healthy diet. Most of the students described that healthy eating was not important to them (Croll et al., 2001).

A study found that the nutritional knowledge of the students was related to their diet and the risk for CVD (Yahia, Brown, Rapley, & Chung, 2016). Students who consumed more than 35% of the calories from fat or daily intake of >300mg cholesterol had low nutrition scores (low nutrition knowledge) than their counterparts. Additionally, nutrition knowledge was negatively correlated with saturated fat and cholesterol intake (Yahia et al., 2016). Previous research showed that females displayed a higher level of nutrition knowledge than males (Livingston, Saafir, & Manuel, 2012). In general, nutrition knowledge plays a crucial role in improving the dietary habits and students feel confident to make healthy food choices when they have appropriate nutrition knowledge (Contento, Koch, Lee, & Calabrese-Barton, 2010).

Recommendations and Intake of Dietary Fat

The recommendations for fats in a 2000Kcal healthy diet is 27g, about 5 teaspoons. Around 20%-35% of the total calories should come from fats is the recommendation. Saturated fats (SF) should account for no more than 10% of the total calories. Some common sources of SF in the American diet are burgers, sandwiches, pizza, taco, rice, pasta, meat, poultry, seafood dishes. It is very important to monitor the fat intake because as per the latest dietary guidelines and current pattern in the U.S., college students consume more than the recommended intake for saturated fats (U.S. Department of Health and Human Services, Centers for Disease Control and Prevention, 2019).

The average intake of cholesterol from the diet is ~0.6g/day while the body synthesizes approximately 1g/day. For an adult consuming 2000 kcal/day, the recommended intake of omega-3 FA is ~1g/day (Stipanuk, 2006). Most of the Americans exceed the recommendations for fat and do not meet the recommended intakes of fruits and vegetables and enough physical activity (U.S. Department of Health and Human Services, Centers for Disease Control and Prevention, 2019).

Diet Quality of College Students

It is widely known that poor diet quality leads to an increased risk of chronic diseases (Papadaki, Hondros, Scott, & Kapsokefalou, 2007). Diet adequacy or diet quality can be assessed by comparing the dietary intake with the established recommendations and guidelines (Waijers, Feskens, & Ocké, 2007). Diet quality indices provide a single score that represents overall diet quality based on current scientific evidence and dietary recommendations. A higher score indicates better diet quality and vice versa (Thorpe, Kestin, Riddell, Keast, & McNaughton, 2013). A decline in diet quality is observed while there is a transition from adolescence to adulthood (Forshee, Richard, & Storey, 2006). Frequent consumption of commercially prepared meals is associated with poor diet quality (Burns, Jackson, Gibbons, & Stoney, 2002).

A study conducted in Balearic Islands analyzed food patterns and physical activity among university students, it was found that there was high consumption of food items which should be avoided, such as red and processed meat, snacks, soft drinks, pastries, sweets, butter, and margarine and their diet quality was found to be low

(Moreno-Gomez et al., 2012). Previous research also showed that consumption of commercially prepared meals was found to be inversely associated with diet quality (French, Story, Neumark-Sztainer, Fulkerson, & Hannan, 2001). Another factor that influenced the quality of diet was participation in meal preparation. Involvement in cooking and less frequent consumption of commercial foods were associated with higher diet quality (Thorpe et al., 2013).

Food Habits and Behavior of College Students

Eating behavior has been an important factor influencing student's weight status. According to the research conducted in universities in the U.S., student did not eat enough fruits and vegetables, and consumed high amounts of fat-rich foods (Silliman, Rodas-Fortier, & Neyman, 2004). Eating fast foods more than three times a week was associated with a higher consumption of fat and added sugars. Students who consumed food brought from home exhibited higher intake of fruits and vegetables and lower intake of fat and added sugars (Pelletier & Laska, 2013). Further, previous studies also showed that there was decreased consumption of bread and vegetables in the first year of college, and increased consumption of alcohol and fat (Butler, Black, Blue, & Gretebeck, 2004). College students who lived away from home for the first time were likely to eat "outside" meals including foods high in fat and calories (Guthrie, Lin, & Frazao, 2002). It has been observed that the students who live with their parents consumed more fruits, vegetables, pulses and fish and the reason for this might be greater involvement of their family in the meal preparation and grocery shopping (Krešić et al., 2009). In contrast, higher consumption of fried and fast foods and lower intake of fruits and vegetables has been shown in the students living away from home (Šatalić, Barić, & Keser, 2007). Besides, alcohol consumption was higher among students living away from their homes as compared to those living with their families (Lau, Quadrel, & Hartman, 1990). A considerable increase of meat (Brown, Dresen, & Eggett, 2005) and decreased intake of protein (Brevard & Ricketts, 1996) had been found in the students living on-campus as compared to their respective counterparts. In a qualitative study, it was found that the students who were more aware and responsible for their meals before going to university were found to have more stable and healthier food choices in college (Cluskey & Grobe, 2009).

Differences in dietary behaviors between sex

There have been differences observed in the dietary habits between male and female university students. Male students were found to have less-healthful eating habits as compared to females. They consumed fast foods frequently (Huang et al., 1994), were less likely to read the nutrition labels (Oakes & Slotterback, 2000), have breakfast, and prepare their own food (Musingo & Wang, 2009). Most studies demonstrated that males consumed more high-fat foods (Wardle et al., 2004). Women were found to consume more fruits and vegetables, men consumed greater amount of fiber, and more servings of fruits and vegetables (Thompson et al., 2005). A review study looked at the barriers of healthy eating and it was found that men perceived healthy eating as less important contributing to their behavior (Wardle et al., 2004). A cross-sectional survey of eating habits reported that male students needed to have a more urgent need to reduce the fat content from their foods while females were required to increase their fiber intake via more consumption of fruits and vegetables (Li et al., 2012). Another study conducted at a university in Saudi Arabia showed that male students were more overweight and obese as compared to female students (Al-Rethaiaa, Fahmy & Al-Shwaiyat, 2010). A survey-based study reported that male students consumed more fat than female students while female's diet consisted less of fibers, fruits and vegetables. Also, female students were found to engage more in healthful eating practices (Li et al., 2012).

Factors Affecting the Food Choices of College Students

The food choices of college students are influenced by numerous factors such as taste, cost, nutritive value, convenience, palatability and weight issues (Glanz et al., 1998). Students tend to eat more fatty foods and fewer fruits and vegetables during their college life due to their changed lifestyle as compared to when they lived with their parents and independent decision making (Murakami, Sasaki, Takahashi, Uenishi, & J.D.S.S, 2011). A study showed that the dietary habits established in the first two years of college life are likely to be continued in the later college years (Driskell et al., 2005).

Stress could be one of the factors having an impact on the food habits of college students because University entrance could be a stressful experience in terms of major life changes like time management, financial stress, assignments, and deadlines (El Ansari, Labeeb, Moseley, Kotb, & El-Houfy, 2013). Evidence suggests that stress alters eating behaviors by choosing the foods with more palatability and energy-dense, especially the ones higher in fat and sugar (Zellnar et al., 2007). Especially, women with relatively more stress were found to consume more calorie-dense foods than the less stressed ones. This relation was not found in males (Mikolajczyk, El Ansari, & Maxwell, 2009). Chronic stress situation is associated with increased exposure to Cortisol which impacts the Brain Reward Pathways (BRP). Cortisol increases BRP sensitivity which in turn triggers the desire to consume high palatability foods (Adam & Epel, 2007). In turn, it produces a positive feeling towards foods high in fat and sugar and stressed people start to relate these foods to the feeling of reward (Zheng, Lenard, Shin, & Berthoud, 2009). A pilot study on college students found that a higher level of perceived stress was associated with uncontrolled and emotional eating. Students with a higher level of stress consumed more frequent fast foods, ready-to-eat snacks and sandwiches (de Oliveira Penaforte, Matta, & Japur, 2016).

Living condition could be another factor for college students in making food choices. Research showed that those living on-campus reported decreased meal frequency, lower intake of fruits, vegetables and dairy (Freedman et al., 2008). In a study conducted in Northern Italy, the majority of the students reported that they have changed their dietary habits while attending university and the change was more prominent in the students living away from home (Lupi et al., 2015). A study showed that adolescents who consumed higher amounts of commercially prepared foods reported low intakes of fruits, vegetables, dietary fiber, vitamins, minerals and higher intakes of energy, fat, meat and confectionery (Murakami et al., 2011). Also, for those who could not cook their meals were more reliable on the pre-prepared and processed foods than those who did cook

(Soliah, Walter, & Antosh, 2006). A study revealed that the students related healthy eating to family meals and something they would not prefer with friends. This reflects that there is an influence of peers and friends on their food habits (Croll et al., 2011).

Lack of access to the food preparation facilities was one of the barriers affecting food choices of college students (LaCaille et al., 2011). Also, poor nutrition education can contribute to increased risk of diet-related diseases (Vidgen & Gallegos, 2014). Additionally, after the nutrition course as an intervention, there was a decline in fast food consumption and students' food cooking skills improved, however, the sample size was really small so it is less likely to be generalized to the whole population (Jones, Robine, & Rathman, 2019).

Campus food outlets provide fast foods like French-fries, pizza, burger regularly and this could contribute to the increased fat intake and weight gain in the freshman year (Niemeier et al., 2006). College meal plans provide prepaid cards which allow the students to pay for a fast-food meal with a swipe. These plans increase their financial access because they do not have to pay out of their pocket and dollars will go further when spent on cheaper meals. Flex dollars, as the additional meal allowances have also been found as a factor affecting the frequency of fast-food consumption (Driskell et al., 2005).

Nutrition label use has been linked to improve the choice of foods from unhealthy to healthy choices, however, only little has been known till date. Individuals who read the nutrition labels frequently tend to think that eating healthy is important than those who do not (Drichoutis, 2005). Other differences are behavioral (individuals who read labels frequently tend to eat more healthy foods) (Pérez-Escamilla, Haldeman, & Gray, 2002). A study conducted on college students at a public university showed that nutrition labels had an impact on the energy intake irrespective of their attitude towards healthy meals (Graham & Laska, 2012).

Peer influence is another big factor affecting the food choices of individuals, especially young adults. At the time of meeting new people, or meeting socially, young adults appear susceptible to the behavior of others. In regard to dietary behavior, they try to match their food choices with family and friends, like the norm of eating pizza after a party, and drinking alcohol before or at a party (Munt et al., 2017). This influence is not limited to face-to-face interactions, but also influenced by social media trends on dietary behaviors. By replicating those behaviors, young adults feel a sense of inclusion, acceptance, and confidence (Burchell, Rettie, & Patel, 2013).

College students find a hard time balancing their academics, work, and social life, which leave them with a lack of time. In order to save time, they engage in frequent snacking, eating quickly as opposed to main meals, ordering take-away, eating fast-foods, or eating while watching TV, working (Celnik, Gillespie, & Lean, 2012). In a pre-post study, majority of the students reported lack of time as a barrier to healthy eating because they did not have time to prepare food, a few of them did not have the equipment to prepare food. They look at healthy eating as a burden because of the busy schedules. These activities contribute to consumption of high-fat foods, which are poor in nutrition and in excess of their energy requirements (Celnik et al., 2012).

The perception of unhealthy diets being cheaper is enhanced by the student's financial instability. A meta-analysis found that a healthy diet, or the one closely related with the recommendations was more expensive by around U.S. $1.50/day (Rao, Afshin, Singh, & Mozaffarian, 2013). To balance finances, money-saving strategies are employed, which includes purchase of convenience or fast-foods that provides taste, satiety, energy at a lower price. Regardless of whether the cost of healthy foods or the cheapness of unhealthy foods is true in reality, the perception of price strongly impacts preference of unhealthy foods (Mhurchu, Cliona, & Ogra, 2007). The affordability of foods is associated with meal choice and foods sold from fast-food outlets tend to contain ingredients which are easily accessible and are cheap, hence, the meals made from them are low in price (Nestle et al., 1998). Pricing of foods is yet another important factor that may contribute indirectly to a higher risk of obesity. For instance, U.S. farm subsidy policies might have caused certain foods in abundance and cheaper, potentially contributing to lower prices and increased consumption of fatty foods (Wallinga, 2010).

College students spend more time on social media than any other activity (Coyne, Padilla-Walker, & Howard, 2013). Social media may be an important factor affecting their food choices. Media and technology have been credited as one of the factors which has changed the perceptions, attitudes, and beliefs about nutrition (Freeland-Graves & Nitzke, 2013). Spending time watching TV, video games, cell phones are conceptualized as sedentary activities that replace time for physical activity and eventually lead to increases in BMI in children and adolescents (Arora et al., 2013). The abdominal weight gain in college students was partially explained by food and beverage consumption while watching TV because they were more likely to consume energy-dense foods with less moderation while eating and watching TV concurrently (Blass et al., 2006). Young adults have turned to social media for seeking nutrition-related information and support (McKinley & Wright, 2014), and this could mislead them because the information on the internet could be sometimes inaccurate, oversimplified, or exaggerated (Freeland-Graves & Nitzke, 2013).

With the changing status of economy, and women being more involved in work, there is a decrease in the skills of young adults for preparing their own food (Blake et al., 2009). They have a lack of skills in planning, shopping, preparation, and cooking of healthy foods because over the past decades, home food consumption and time spent preparing food have declined considerably (Anderson, Butcher, & Levine, 2003). Other factors include failure to realize the long-term benefits and/or drawbacks of following a healthy/unhealthy diet during young adulthood. They prioritize social inclusion, taste, cheapness over long-term consequences of health (Munt et al., 2017).

Other factors such as campus dining services may also affect their dietary intake. The campus food outlets can compete with fast-food restaurants and serve energy-dense options like pizza, burgers, fries regularly which highly impact the diet of the students (Niemeier et al., 2006). Nearly half of the students bought food from campus resources more than three times a week according to a cross-sectional health and wellness study (Pelletier & Laska, 2013). A study reported that the most common reason for not eating healthy was the limited availability of healthy foods within the dining facility (Peterson, Duncan, Null, Roth, & gill, 2010). According to the results of a cross-sectional study,

22% of the students reported purchasing fast foods from McDonald's, Burger King, Hardee's more than three times a week.

Weight gain is not only affected by dietary factors, but certain medications also contribute to rapid weight gain. These medications include psychotropic medications, diabetic treatments, anti-hypertensives, steroid hormones, and contraceptives to name a few (Aronne, Nelinson, & Lillo, 2009). Some of the most widely prescribed classes of drugs can cause significant weight gain, which supports the hypothesis that drug-induced weight gain is contributing to the obesity epidemic. Moreover, sleep debt has also been linked to an increase in weight. Some studies demonstrated that hours of sleep per night were negatively correlated to the BMI (Gangwisch, Malaspina, Boden-Albala, & Heymsfield, 2005) while sleep restriction was shown to increase hunger and appetite (Spiegel, Tasali, Penev, & Van Cauter, 2004).

Interventions for the Improvement of Nutrition Knowledge and Food Choices

Food habits that are cultivated in college life are likely to be continued for most of life (Ha & Caine-Bish, 2011). Meal skipping, fast food consumption, unhealthy dieting are common habits during college life which would make them vulnerable to increased risk of various diseases such as obesity, Diabetes, Osteoporosis, CVD and Cancer in the later part of life (Lua & Wan Putri Elena, 2012). Various interventions have been conducted in the past in the effort to improve the nutrition knowledge and behavior of college students some of which include in-person interaction, online or through Point-Of-Purchase (POP) messages.

Research has shown that college students consume only about 0.7 servings of whole-grain products per day which is inadequate for their daily requirements (Rose, Hosig, Davy, Serrano, & Davis, 2007). As previously researched, the average student consumes about 1 serving of fruit, 1.5 servings of vegetables and 0.5 servings of low-fat dairy (Poddar et al., 2009). A study showed an increased consumption of whole-grains after a nutrition course intervention focusing on disease prevention (Ha & Caine-Bish, 2011). Another web-based intervention through e-mail, messages increased self-efficacy in the students and showed increased dairy consumption. However, this study was short-term hence, long-term research is required to show whether there is sustainability of the newly improved dietary habits (Poddar et al., 2009). A longitudinal study conducted at a large mid-western public university included a class-based nutrition intervention, lectures and interactions. The students decreased the consumption of soft-drinks and increased the milk intake, however, more than half of the students were females (Ha, Caine-Bish, Holloman, & Lowry-Gordon, 2009).

Cooking classes could be one such innovative intervention to help the students improve their cooking skills to take care of their nutritional status (Levy & Auld, 2004). The results also show that female students are relatively motivated as compared to male counterparts (Ha et al., 2009). Female students are more likely to take part in weight-related programs as they are more concerned about their shape. Taken together, many in-person and online interventions improved nutrition knowledge, awareness, and readiness to develop healthy dietary habits among college students. A pilot study considered Mobile MyPlate as the tool to provide nutrition education to the students accompanied by regular text messaging. As a result, most of the participants found text messaging helpful to focus on their health (Brown, O'Connor, & Savaiano, 2014). A study conducted in Sweden included face-to-face counseling session followed by providing them with self-help materials covering physical activity, diet, and weight control, there were significant results observed on their weight and BMI after 12 months of intervention (Eiben & Lissner, 2006).

Overweight students are at a greater risk of certain diseases in later life. As students often turn to the internet for health information, an internet-based obesity program was carried out involving 320 undergraduate students. It lowered stress and improved healthy eating behaviors (LaChausse, 2012). Also, educating the students on portion sizes would help further in advancing the level of nutrition education. According to the study that included the nutrition module as their intervention, most of the students found it helpful and learned new information on budget-friendly food preparation. They reported being unaware of the calories and fat that they consumed before the intervention (Kicklighter, Koonce, Rosenbloom, & Commander, 2010).

Traffic light labels classify foods and beverages from green (most healthy), to red (lease healthy) and provide quick information at the point of sale (Thorndike et al., 2012). A study conducted in 2010 at a hospital cafeteria concluded that the use of traffic light label increased the purchase of healthy foods and decreased buying of unhealthy items (Thorndike et al., 2012). Another study conducted at college cafeteria found that labels were well received by the students and most of them found the labels helpful. Also, athletes were more likely to want nutrition information on labels (Seward, Block, & Chatterjee, 2016).

Food prepared away from home is generally high in saturated fat and calories. A culinary nutrition course helped the students to improve cooking practices as well as gain confidence to take charge of their health (Jones et al., 2019). On the other hand, dietary habits and nutrition knowledge has been shown to improve significantly by various interactions and interventions (Lua & Wan Putri Elena, 2012). Interventions like a basic nutrition course improved whole-grain intake (Ha & Caine-Bish, 2011); nutrition education and supplementation significantly reduced body weight, body fat, waist-hip ratio and BMI in Korean female college students (You, Sung, & Chang, 2009); a combination of lectures and laboratory exercises resulted into prevention of weight gain in at-risk first-year female students (Matvienko, Lewis, & Schafer, 2001). However, there is a lack of long-term studies in Nutrition education interventions to conclude that the subjects sustain the newly improved dietary habits for a longer period (Kelly, Mazzeo, & Bean, 2013).

CHAPTER III

METHODS

The purpose of this study was to measure the differences between fat-related diet habits in college students of varying BMI statuses and sex at a large mid-western public university. It was a quantitative research with cross-sectional design (online survey). The independent variables for this study were the BMI statuses categorized into underweight, normal, overweight, obese, and sex (males and females). The dependent variable was their dietary habits related to fat. The hypotheses for the study were that there were differences in the fat-related diet habits of college students between different BMI statuses and sex. For statistical analyses, a multifactorial (4x2) ANOVA was used. An approval for this study from the Institutional Review Board (IRB) had been obtained (IRB number: 20-010).

Sample

This study used convenience sampling. The inclusion criteria for the study were the following: participant must be enrolled in any course at Kent State University; must be between 18-25 years of age and must be either male or female in sex. The exclusion criteria for the study were: any other gender than male or female, and less than 18 years/more than 25 years in age. The weight and the height were self-reported by the participants.

Survey

The data was collected via a survey which included filling out a questionnaire. An online Fat-related Diet Habits Questionnaire (Kristal et al., 1990) was used as the measurement tool. The original questionnaire was used and all parts of the questionnaire (Appendix A) were in English language. It was available to the subjects online using Qualtrics and had two main parts.

Part-1

The first part included five demographic questions: age (years), sex (male/female/other), weight (kg or lbs), height (feet or inches), and living condition (on-campus off-campus).

Part-2

The second part included questions related to the frequency of consuming certain foods in the past month which were answered using Likert scale (usually, often, sometimes, rarely/never). There were 22 questions in this part, each question was related to either of the five factors: Substitution, modifying meat, avoid frying, replacement, and avoid fat. The first factor, substitution, consisted of seven questions, and were related to the substitution of the full-fat products to low-fat or non-fat alternatives. The second factor, modifying meat, consisted of three questions, and were related to how often they removed the skin before eating the chicken or trimmed all the visible fat from the red meat. The third factor, avoid frying, consisted of four questions, and included the frequency of fried options such as French fries, hash-browns instead of the boiled or baked options. The fourth factor, replacement, consisted of three questions, and they were related to the replacement of fat-rich foods with healthier options such as fruits and vegetables. The last factor, avoid fat, consisted of two questions, and included adding extra fat to the foods.

Procedures

The process began with the selection of the questionnaire. A total of 10 questionnaires were reviewed and fat-related diet habits questionnaire was finalized. Next, a request of IRB (Institutional Review Board) approval was obtained before the collection of data. Data collection was done by publishing online questionnaire to target population by email. The email addresses of the participants were provided by the office of Registrar. An email with the description of the survey (Appendix B) to explain the purpose of this research and to provide contact person for the participants if they have questions or any concern was sent to the subjects. The link to access the survey was only provided once in order to avoid duplication of data from the same subject. Participation in the study was anonymous and voluntary with no compensation given and this term was stated on electronic consent (Appendix C) at the beginning of the questionnaire. By clicking the electronic consent, participants agreed on terms given and they were at least 18 years of age. A reminder email was sent to them after one week to complete the survey. Once they answered the last question, they were asked to hit submit and then clicked out of the survey. After two weeks of data collection process, all data was returned via Qualtrics XM and was analyzed statistically with SPSS statistics software version 25.0.

Data Analysis

All the data was collected via Qualtrics and analyzed with several methods. For demographic data, summarization of the mean frequencies and standard deviation was provided in simple tabulation. For the four-point Likert scale on each question, every response recorded was scored as following: "Usually" valued as four, "Often" as three, "Sometimes" as two and "Rarely/Never" as one. From all 22 questions, the minimum possible score was 1 and the maximum possible score was 4. Lower scores indicated less consumption of fatty foods while higher scores demonstrated higher and more frequent consumption of foods rich in fat. For scoring, firstly, the 22 questions were divided into five factors as Substitution (factor 1), Modify meat (factor 2), Avoid frying (factor 3), Replacement (factor 4), and Avoid fat (factor 5). The final score was calculated by adding up the average means of all the five sub-scales and dividing it by five to get a final summary score. Participants who completed less than 90% of the questionnaire and/or who chose the option "wish not to specify" for sex category was excluded from statistical analysis because this study looked at the differences between males and females. Finally, to test hypotheses, multifactorial (two-way) ANOVA (Analysis of Variance) was used. The two independent variables were BMI statuses (kg/m^2): underweight (<18.5), normal (18.5 - <25), overweight (25 - <30), obese (≥ 30) and sex (male/female). The weight and height were self-reported by the participants. The dependent variable was their fat-related diet habits. The dependent variable was their fat-related diet habits. The statistical methods looked at the differences in fat-related diet habits between males and females as well as between different BMI ranges. All results were considered significant at $p \leq 0.05$.

CHAPTER IV

JOURNAL ARTICLE

Introduction

Obesity continues to be a major public health concern around the globe over decades and specifically in the U.S. According to a report from 1998-2008, more than 68% of the U.S. adults were overweight, and 35% were obese (Flegal, Caroll, Ogden, & Curtin, 2010). This poses severe health risks and a huge economic burden on society because overweight and obesity lead to chronic diseases such as hypertension, type 2 diabetes, cardiovascular diseases, cancer and premature death (Report of a Joint WHO/FAO expert consultation, 2003).

Monitoring the fat intake during the transition from adolescence to young adulthood is crucial because it is found to be a challenging period, there are many lifestyle and dietary changes involved (Lassi, Moin, & Bhutta, 2017). There is often increased consumption of fast-foods and processed foods and decreased consumption of fruits and vegetables because they start making independent food choices (Neumark-Sztainer et al., 2011). There are nationally recognized guidelines given by The Academy of Nutrition and Dietetics for grains, protein, fruits, vegetables, dairy, fats/oils, added sugars, and physical activity, despite the available guidelines, nutritional problems continue to be prevalent in college students (U.S. Department of Health and Human Services, Centers for Disease Control and Prevention, 2019).

The recommendations for fats in a 2000Kcal healthy diet for adults is 27g, about 5 teaspoons. Around 20%-35% of the total calories should come from fats is the recommendation. The average intake of oils in the US by young adults is 35-40g per day (U.S. Department of Health and Human Services, Centers for Disease Control and Prevention, 2019). Saturated fats (SF) should account for no more than 10% of the total calories. Some common sources of SF in the American diet are burgers, sandwiches, pizza, taco, rice, pasta, meat, poultry, seafood dishes (U.S. Department of Health and Human Services, Centers for Disease Control and Prevention, 2019). It is very important to monitor the fat intake because as per the latest dietary guidelines and current pattern in the U.S., college students consume more than the recommended intake for saturated fats (U.S. Department of Health and Human Services, Centers for Disease Control and Prevention, 2019).

Their food choices are influenced by several factors including taste, cost, nutritive value, convenience, palatability and weight issues (Glanz, Basil, Maibach, Goldberg, & Snyder, 1998), stress (Zellnar, Saito, & Gonzalez, 2007), living condition (Freedman, 2010), access to the food preparation facilities (LaCaille, Dauner, Krambeer, & Pederson, 2011), nutrition education (Vidgen & Gallegos, 2014), campus food outlets (Niemeier, Raynor, Lloyd-Richardson, Rogers, & Wing, 2006), peer influence (Munt, Patridge, & Allman-Farinelli, 2017), and social media (Freeland-Graves & Nitzke, 2013). Another major factor affecting their dietary habits is portion sizes. They have shown to affect weight because restaurants serve large portion sizes for fatty foods (Diliberti, Bordi, Conklin, Roe, & Rolls, 2004). Physical activity is another important factor influencing obesity in college students. More than 60% of college students do not engage in moderate or vigorous exercise (National College Health Assessment 2: Reference Group Executive Summary 2011).

There have been differences observed in the dietary habits between male and female university students. Male students were found to have less healthy eating habits as compared to females. They consumed fast foods frequently (Huang, Song, Schemmel, & Hoerr, 1994), were less likely to read the nutrition labels (Oakes & Slotterback, 2000), have breakfast, and prepare their food (Musingo & Wang, 2009). A survey-based study reported that male students consumed more fat than female students while female's diets consisted less of fibers, fruits, and vegetables. Also, female students were found to engage more in healthful eating practices (Li et al., 2012).

Various interventions have been conducted in the past in the effort to improve the nutrition knowledge and behavior of college students some of which include in-person interaction, online or through Point-Of-Purchase (POP) messages. Nutrition course (Ha & Caine-Bish, 2011), cooking demonstrations (Levy & Auld, 2004), use of traffic light labels (Thorndike, Sonnenberg, Riis, Barraclough, & Levy, 2012) were some of the interventions found effective in improving their nutrition knowledge as well as food choices. However, there is a lack of long-term studies to observe the change or improvement in their food choices or dietary habits. This study looked at the differences in fat-related diet habits of college students at a large mid-western public university between sex and varying BMI statuses. BMI is a useful tool to measure overweight and obesity. It is an estimate of the fat mass in the body. Higher the BMI, the higher is the risk of chronic diseases. There have been constant increases in weight and BMI during college life and hence, it is very important to monitor the BMI during young adulthood coupled with the fat intake (Gropper, Simmons, Connell, & Ulrich, 2012). It was hypothesized that there were differences between both the sex and the BMI categories.

Methodology

The purpose of this study was to measure the differences between fat-related diet habits in college students of varying BMI statuses and sex at a large mid-western university. It was a quantitative research with cross-sectional design (online survey). The independent variables for this study were the BMI statuses categorized into underweight, normal, overweight, obese, and sex (males and females). The dependent variable was their dietary habits related to fat. The hypotheses for the study were that there were differences in the fat-related diet habits of college students between different BMI statuses and sex. Approval for this study from the Institutional Review Board (IRB) had been obtained (IRB number: 20-010).

Sample

The sampling method used for this study was convenience sampling. The inclusion criteria for the participant, were the following: the subject must be enrolled in any course at Kent State University; must be between 18-25 years of age and must be either male or female in sex.

Survey

The data was collected via a survey which included filling out a questionnaire. An online Fat-related Diet Habits Questionnaire (Kristal, Shattuck & Henry, 1990) was used as the measurement tool. The original questionnaire was used, and all parts of the questionnaire were in the English language. It was available to the subjects online using Qualtrics and had two main parts.

Part-1: The first part included five demographic questions: age (years), sex (male/female/other), weight (kg or lbs), height (feet or inches), and living conditions (on-campus off-campus). The weight and height were self-reported by the participants.

Part-2: The second part included questions related to the frequency of consuming certain foods in the past month which were answered using a Likert scale (usually, often, sometimes, rarely/never). There were 22 questions in this part, each question was related to either of the five factors: Substitution, modifying meat, avoid frying, replacement, and avoid fat. The first factor, substitution, consisted of seven questions, and were related to the substitution of the full-fat products to low-fat or non-fat alternatives. The second factor, modifying meat, consisted of three questions, and were related to how often they removed the skin before eating the chicken or trimmed all the visible fat from the red meat. The third factor, avoid frying, consisted of four questions, and included the frequency of fried options such as French fries, hash-browns instead of the boiled or baked options. The fourth factor, replacement, consisted of three questions, and they were related to the replacement of fat-rich foods with healthier options such as fruits and vegetables. The last factor, avoid fat, consisted of two questions, and included adding extra fat to the foods.

Procedures

The procedures for this study were started with the selection of a validated questionnaire. A total of 10 questionnaires were reviewed and a fat-related diet habits questionnaire was finalized. Next, a request for IRB (Institutional Review Board) approval was obtained before the collection of data. Data collection was done by publishing an online questionnaire to the target population by email. The email addresses of the participants were provided by the office of Registrar. An email with the description of the survey to explain the purpose of this research and to provide a contact person for the participants if they have questions or any concern was sent to the subjects. The link to access the survey was only provided once to avoid duplication of data from the same subject. Participation in the study was anonymous and voluntary with no compensation given and this term was stated on electronic consent at the beginning of the questionnaire. By clicking the electronic consent, participants agreed on terms given and they were at least 18 years of age. A reminder email was sent to them after one week to complete the survey. Once they answered the last question, they were asked to hit submit and then clicked out of the survey. After two weeks of the data collection process, all data was returned via Qualtrics XM and was analyzed statistically with SPSS statistics software version 25.0.

Data Analysis

All the data was collected via Qualtrics and analyzed with several methods. For demographic data, a summarization of the mean frequencies and standard deviation was provided in the simple tabulation. For the four-point Likert scale on each question, every response recorded was scored as follows: "Usually" valued as four, "Often" as three, "Sometimes" as two and "Rarely/Never" as one. From all 22 questions, the minimum possible score was 1 and the maximum possible score was 4. Lower scores indicated less consumption of fatty foods while higher scores demonstrated higher and more frequent consumption of foods rich in fat. For the scoring, firstly, the 22 questions were divided into five factors as Substitution (factor 1), Modify meat (factor 2), Avoid frying (factor 3), Replacement (factor 4), and Avoid fat (factor 5). Each factor score was obtained by adding up the scores of individual questions followed by dividing it by the number of questions answered. Finally, the total score was obtained by adding up the average means of all the five sub-scales and dividing it by five to get a final summary score. Participants who completed less than 90% of the questionnaire and/or who chose the option "wish not to specify" for the sex category were excluded from statistical analysis because this study looked at the differences between males and females. Finally, to test the hypotheses, multifactorial (two-way) ANOVA was used. The two independent variables were BMI statuses (kg/m^2): underweight (<18.5), normal ($18.5 - <25$), overweight ($25 - <30$), obese (≥ 30) and sex (Male/Female). The weight and height were self-reported by the participants. The dependent variable was their fat-related diet habits. The statistical methods looked at the differences in fat-related diet habits between males and females as well as between different BMI ranges. All results were considered significant at $p \leq 0.05$.

Results

The response rate for this study was 5%. The total number of emails sent out were 24,310, out of which 1248 responses were recorded. Out of this number, 466 participants were excluded from the sample based on invalid age or they completed less than 90% of the questionnaire. Furthermore, 10 were excluded because they were outliers, they presented unrealistic data such as 10 feet tall and weighing about 60 lbs. Lastly, eight participants were excluded because they answered other/not to specify for the sex question. Therefore, the total number of participants used in the data analysis were 764 subjects.

Demographics

Table 1 represents the demographic distribution between the sex, BMI categories, their age, and living situation. Most of the participants were females (81.4%). Among the four BMI categories, 6.7% of the total participants were underweight (<18.5), 56.8% were under normal BMI range (18.5-<25), 20.8% were overweight (25-<30), and 15.7% were obese (≥30). Nearly half of the participants reported living off-campus without parents (44.3%), 34.6% of the subjects lived on-campus, and 21.1% lived off-campus with their parents. Maximum number of the participants were aged between 18-20 years old.

Table 1
The demographic information of the college students at a large mid-western university

Variable	Category	n
Sex	Male	142
	Female	622
BMI	Underweight	51
	Normal	434
	Overweight	159
	Obese	120
Living condition	On-campus	267
	Off-campus with parents	163
	Off-campus apartment (without parents)	342

A four-point Likert scale was used for scoring, wherein, "always=1", "often=2", "sometimes=3", and "rarely/never=4".

Sex Differences Between the Fat-Related Dietary Patterns

Table 2 depicts the sex differences in the fat-related diet habits of college students at a large mid-western university. The summary scores of the sample represented that most of the participants consumed fat-rich foods moderately and consuming the fatty foods "always" was not reported by them. The differences in the dietary habits related to consumption of fatty foods were not significant between sex ($p= 0.48$), or between the BMI categories ($p = 0.31$).

For the first sub-scale, males and females reported following a similar pattern of substituting full-fat products with low-fat or non-fat alternatives sometimes. These included substituting full-fat dressing, milk, cheese, mayonnaise with low-fat or non-fat alternatives. They made their cookies, cakes, and pies with less butter or fat, and used the cooking spray for sautéing instead of using fat "sometimes". However, there were no significant differences found in the fat substitution habits between males and females ($p = 0.55$).

For the second sub-scale, there were small differences found between males and females, with the means and standard deviations of $2.54 \pm .94$ and $2.44 \pm .93$ respectively. The questions included removing the skin before eating the chicken, trimmed all the visible fat from red meat, and ate extra lean ground meat. They reported that some of them modified the form of meat that they consumed sometimes and the other modified it less often. There were no significant differences found in the habits related to modifying meat between males and females ($p = 0.23$)

For the third sub-scale, there were similar patterns observed between both the sex. The questions were related to fried foods and these foods included fried chicken, fried fish, fried vegetables, and fried potatoes like French fries or hash-browns. Both, males and females reported consuming fried foods often. There were no significant differences found in the fat-related diet habits between males and females ($p = 0.12$).

For the fourth sub-scale, small differences were reported in the dietary habits related to the replacement of the foods between males and females. Both, males and females replaced fat-rich foods with healthier options sometimes. This scale included having a vegetarian meal without any meat, replacing any fruit as a dessert, and replacing raw vegetables or fruits as a snack between meals. However, these differences were not significant ($p = 0.08$).

For the fifth sub-scale, there were small differences observed between the dietary habits related to adding extra fat to their foods between males and females, with them adding the fat often to sometimes. The questions took into consideration the frequency of adding an extra fat source in the food. It included consuming spaghetti or noodles without adding meat, add butter or other fat to cooked vegetables, consuming baked or boiled potatoes without adding fat or sour cream, and eating bread rolls, muffins, rolls without adding fat. However, there were no significant differences found in the habits related to replacement of the foods between sex ($p = 0.18$).

Table 2
Sex differences in the fat-related diet habits of college students at a large mid-western university including the summary score and the individual scores for the sub-scales

Scale	Sex	n	Mean ± Standard Deviation
Summary score	Male	142	2.45 ± .54
	Female	764	2.44 ± .52
Sub-scale 1: substitution	Male	141	3.00 ± .79
	Female	620	3.04 ± .72
Sub-scale 2: modifying meat	Male	127	2.54 ± .94
	Female	541	2.44 ± .93
Sub-scale 3: avoid frying	Male	142	1.94 ± .63
	Female	619	1.84 ± .66
Sub-scale 4: replacement	Male	135	2.81 ± .83
	Female	617	2.65 ± .74
Sub-scale 5: avoid fat	Male	142	2.40 ± .73
	Female	620	2.56 ± .67

A four-point Likert scale was used for scoring, wherein, “always=1”, “often=2”, “sometimes=3”, and “rarely/never=4”.

Table 3
Differences in the fat-related diet habits between the BMI categories of college students at a large mid-western university including the summary scores and the individual scores for the five sub-scales

Scale	BMI category	n	Mean ± Standard Deviation
Summary score	Underweight	51	2.36 ± .61
	Normal	434	2.43 ± .52
	Overweight	159	2.39 ± .52
	Obese	120	2.56 ± .44
	Total	764	2.44 ± .52
Sub-scale 1: substitution	Underweight	50	3.01 ± .82
	Normal	433	3.05 ± .71
	Overweight	159	3.00 ± .80
	Obese	119	3.03 ± .67
	Total	761	3.03 ± .73
Sub-scale 2: modifying meat	Underweight	43	2.40 ± .88
	Normal	373	2.45 ± .94
	Overweight	139	2.38 ± .97
	Obese	113	2.59 ± .90
	Total	668	2.46 ± .94
Sub-scale 3: avoid frying	Underweight	51	1.88 ± .72
	Normal	431	1.86 ± .67
	Overweight	159	1.84 ± .65
	Obese	120	1.88 ± .58
	Total	761	1.86 ± .66
Sub-scale 4: replacement	Underweight	50	2.60 ± .85
	Normal	431	2.64 ± .74
	Overweight	154	2.65 ± .79
	Obese	117	2.90 ± .70
	Total	752	2.68 ± .76
Sub-scale 5: avoid fat	Underweight	50	2.44 ± .67
	Normal	433	2.54 ± .69
	Overweight	159	2.46 ± .71
	Obese	120	2.63 ± .65
	Total	762	2.53 ± .69

A four-point Likert scale was used for scoring, wherein, “always=1”, “often=2”, “sometimes=3”, and “rarely/never=4”.

Differences in the Dietary Habits Related to Fat Between Varying BMI Statuses

Table 3 represents the differences in the fat-related diet habits between the four BMI categories: underweight, normal, overweight, and obese. For the summary score, it was found that they consumed fatty foods moderately, all the responses recorded were between "often" and "sometimes". There were small differences observed between their habits with respect to the five sub-scales. However, these differences were not significant except for sub-scale 4: replacement. It was found that those individuals who were in the underweight or normal category for the BMI, replaced the fat-rich foods with healthier alternatives more often than the obese individuals. The difference between the BMI categories for this sub-scale was found to be significant ($p = 0.01$).

Discussion

The primary purpose of this study was to look at the differences in fat-related diet habits of college students between sex and varying BMI statuses at a large mid-western public university. The results showed that there were no significant differences in the dietary habits related to fat between males and females, and between different BMI statuses, so the hypotheses were rejected. The overall habits were similar between males and females with different BMI statuses. The maximum responses recorded were either "often" or "sometimes" in terms of substitution of full-fat products with low-fat/non-fat alternatives, avoiding fried foods, adding an extra source of fat, removing the skin and trimming all the visible fat from the meat, and replacing fruits and vegetables instead of fat-rich food items.

The 2015-2020 Dietary Guidelines (U.S. Department of Health and Human Services, Centers for Disease Control and Prevention, 2019) for Americans recommend that the consumption of oils/fats in a 2000Kcal diet must be limited to five teaspoons (27g). Saturated fat (SF) should account for no more than 10% of the total calories. It is very important to monitor the fat intake because as per the current pattern in the US, college students consume more than the recommended intake for saturated fats (U.S. Department of Health and Human Services, Centers for Disease Control and Prevention, 2019). In this study, fat-related dietary habits were expected to be different significantly with varying BMI statuses and between sex. However, that was not the case. Other factors likely play a more important role in influencing their food habits. According to a review article, it was found that young adults presented a unique challenge to maintain healthy habits and dietary patterns. These habits were influenced by factors such as time, cost, living conditions, social media, physical activity, etc. (Glanz et al., 1998).

The current study showed different results than the previous literature. It has been noted that college students have a high consumption of fatty foods. They also reported a low intake of fruits and vegetables and a high intake of high-fat, high-calorie foods (Brevard & Ricketts, 1996). In this study, it cannot be ignored that none of the data represented that the participants consumed foods rich in fat in high amounts. All the participants reported that they consumed moderate fat-rich foods and replaced them with healthier foods occasionally. There has been a rigorous awareness about obesity, especially in America for a decade now, and this can be added to the existing literature as a starting point of the improvement in the health status of young adults. This can be due to several factors, many of the restaurants, campus food-outlets, and dining halls provide nutrition labels to help the customers choose a healthier option. Moreover, a study done in the past showed that interventions like nutrition food label use improved the food intake of college students (Graham & Laska, 2012). This could be a factor that played a role in improving their knowledge and choice of the foods that they eat regularly.

This study found significant differences between the replacement of the fatty foods with the healthier foods among the various BMI categories. Obese individuals were found to replace foods less often than those in the underweight or normal range for the BMI. This suggests that overweight and obese individuals are at a greater risk for becoming obese and consume fat-rich foods more frequently. However, the direct link between BMI and fat intake has not been researched much, most of the studies considered weight change or weight change coupled with BMI (Gropper et al., 2012) (Racette et al., 2005) (Pope, Hansen, & Harvey, 2016). So, it is hard to compare the findings with the current study. Moreover, the limitation of using BMI as a tool is that it could underestimate or overestimate the nutritional status. For instance, a person who works out heavily might weigh more because of the lean body mass that he gained but could be overweight according to the BMI classification. Likewise, a person could be tall, weigh less, and still be healthy, however, BMI classification could consider him as underweight. so, the BMI distribution in this study could have affected the outcome.

The current study found similar results with small differences in their fat-related habits between various statuses of BMI as well as between the sex. Their responses were quite close in terms of the four-point Likert scale answers. The majority of them answered “often” or “sometimes”, and the two extremities, “always” and “rarely/never” were the least chosen options overall. Past research study showed that there were significant gains in weight and BMI have been observed throughout the four years of college and one of the main factors influencing this weight change was the fat consumption of young adults (Pope et al., 2016). One of the studies also reported that those who are overweight or obese are more likely to under-report their intake than those of a healthy weight. They also found that individuals aged 19-29 years, especially women are likely to under-report (Kye et al., 2014). The fact that the information was self-reported, there are high chances that many of the participants presented inaccurate information which eventually affected the outcomes of the study.

A research study showed that men were less likely than women to follow healthy eating, they were also found to perceive healthy eating as important than women. Also, diet and weight have been traditionally a part of a woman’s life (Munt et al., 2017). Research also showed that females were more concerned about how they looked, and their appearance and were more likely to have weight concerns (Peterson, Grippo & Tantleff-Dunn, 2008). In line with the literature, this study found some differences between the males and females, however, these differences were not significant.

Limitations

The results that this study found, could be due to several factors. Firstly, the results of this study were based on conducting a survey by filling out an online questionnaire. Often with online tools, there is under-reporting or over-reporting of their habits and due to this, their actual habits might have been missed. Secondly, it was a very short period of data collection (two weeks), which could be insufficient to analyze the participants' dietary habits. Thirdly, the results could not be necessarily generalizable because it involves the students from only one campus of a university, a larger sample size could give different results. Next, there was unequal distribution of the sample observed with nearly 85% female participants and only a small number of male participants. It is possible that female students may have been more interested in research studies related to health and weight issues than males. Moreover, a kind of questionnaire used may not estimate their fat intake most accurately and it included only the fat intake of last month, which may or may not be remembered properly and could lead to negligence and vague answers in the survey. A more detailed body measurement tool could also be used to differentiate muscle mass from fat mass in future studies to overcome this limitation. Lastly, convenience sampling may also have impacted the results of this study.

Implications

This study had interesting results in terms of the frequency of consumption of fat-rich foods. There was no data reported portraying very high frequency of consuming fat-rich foods which the literature shows. This could be the turning point to study this population further. On one hand, there have been rises in the obesity rates constantly, but there have also been increases in nutrition knowledge and health awareness among young adults and this might be the reason for the results of this study. This might be the evidence that there is increased awareness among college students and their dietary habits are improved as compared to previous years. Future researchers could use this study as a reference to further evaluate the improvement in their fat consumption. A more detailed method of assessing their dietary fat intake could be used such as 24-hour dietary recall, 3-day food logs, dietary recalls from one whole week, which would more accurately estimate their fat intake. Also, a combination of tools and questionnaires could be beneficial to have an idea about their routine dietary habits. Further, a balance in the male and female population could also help in assessing and generalizing the results.

The current study can be useful to future researchers to track and monitor the change and improvement in their dietary routine by closely looking at the factors affecting their nutritional health. They can also include other food groups to have an overall and detailed dietary analysis. Parameters related to physical activity can also be combined with the dietary analysis to make the most out of the available data. Along with collecting their dietary data, an intervention can be done to have and exact idea about the change in their dietary habits and behavior pre- and post the intervention. This intervention can be a seminar, an online or in-person course, a demonstration, or an individual counseling. Dietitians can step forward to continue spreading awareness and educating about the long-term health consequences of not adhering to the recommended guidelines for dietary habits and physical activity. Health care providers need to be intentional in evaluating the health behaviors of this age group and providing appropriate education to improve health behaviors for optimum health outcomes and wellness.

Conclusions

This study shows that there is no significant difference observed between fat-related diet habits of college students between males and females, and between varying BMI statuses. However, it also provides evidence of improvement in the nutritional status and dietary habits related to fat for young adults. Far from exhausting the discussion on this issue and considering that college students are particularly vulnerable when it comes to dietary intake, especially fat intake, it is worthwhile to highlight the importance of the studies that showed significant results and explore deeper in this issue.

CPSIA information can be obtained
at www.ICGtesting.com
Printed in the USA
LVHW020015280423
745413LV00009B/260

9 781805 281245